Better Than New

Better Than New

Sally Barnes

Two Harbors Press

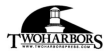

Two Harbors Press
212 3rd Avenue North, Suite 290
Minneapolis, MN 55401
612.455.2293
www.TwoHarborsPress.com

ISBN-13: 978-1-936401-24-6
LCCN: 2011920035

Distributed by Itasca Books
Illustrations by Robert Rafn
Author photo by www.reneelynnphotography.com.
Cover Design and Typeset by Kyle Wyatt

Printed in the United States of America

Steps of My Story

List of Illustrations

For *all* my sisters.

Acknowledgements

There are so many people that made a difference for me as I faced this life-changing experience. Several were new to me, others were from my past with friendships renewed, and of course many were my dear family and long-standing close friends.

Honestly, despite the news of breast cancer, I see myself as quite a lucky person. Blessed with a love of life, laughter, and a reasonable amount of joy, I am sure this is but a chapter in my multi-faceted story.

My sisters and friends gave me the "glamour girl" title long ago as I hold hair, makeup, fashion, and style as key ingredients in my life.

In this book, the names of those who touched me so deeply have been changed or abbreviated to protect their privacy. I am not certain any of them is interested in the spotlight.

What I wish for you, the reader—whether a cancer sister, family member, supportive friend, or just an interested party—is that you will be as blessed as I am to know you are deeply loved.

The most important thing to remember is this:

You are stronger than you think you are.

You can do this.

Foreword

My story began in a most unusual way. And, as a nurse who works for a high-tech medical equipment company I assumed there would be little to surprise me once I chose my path of treatment. This was not the case. Many things surprised me. Even an insider has a lot to learn.

So as I tell my story, I will also show you what I experienced, using diagrams (photos are too scary and, frankly, I am much too modest) and simple, non-medical language combined with (hopefully) a small element of humor to lighten things up a little bit. I have included suggestions as to what to wear, what to prepare, and what little things can make this experience easier.

This book is brief by design. A newly diagnosed breast cancer patient is thrown into what most would agree is crisis mode. Hearing things for the first time, remembering things, and understanding all of the new jargon is a real struggle. Attention spans are shortened and emotions run high.

"Better than New" was my repeated mantra to my dear mother, whom I wanted to reassure the end result of this nightmare would be worth the trouble. I was going to be absolutely lovely. Breast reconstruction medicine has advanced to where women no longer need to fear disfigurement and shame. The results are truly incredible.

I am in no way offering medical advice or recommending this as the best or only treatment option, as I am not qualified to do so. Only your doctors can help you reach this most personal of decisions.

A very important thing to remember is this:

This is your body, your life, your choice.

Be true to yourself.

Anything but Routine:

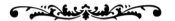

The Photo Shoot. And No Lump?

Well I'd like to boast that I always did all the right things in life, but that isn't true exactly. But, really, is it for anybody? What I can tell you is I never smoked (anything), did drugs, or had a drinking issue. Well, not since college anyway . . . unless you count those annual sales meetings where a bit of excess often leads to much dancing.

I ate healthy foods and was pretty good at exercising on a regular basis I've been told I did nothing to bring this about and that made me feel better. But really, unless you have unlucky genes there isn't an explanation for breast cancer; better not to dwell on that which we cannot change.

Remember this is not your fault.

You are still fabulous!

So here is the weird part. I was overdue for my annual mammogram by a few months, and having debated going on an every-other-year schedule, it was the farthest thing from my mind. Then the itching began, and it was bad—and on both breasts.

Thinking surely it was hormonal, after ruling out any new soaps or perfumes in my bath, I tried to ignore it. But it would not be denied; it was keeping me up at night and, overall, kind of driving me nuts. Then, while reading one of my favorite women's magazines, I found an article on breast cancer that mentioned itching as a sign of the disease. That startled me, and though I didn't have a rash (and it was on both sides) I figured it was a sign to get my appointment scheduled.

Signs are everywhere . . . you only have to look.

Pay attention to them . . . they are there to protect you.

I had no lump, nothing doctors or myself could feel.

So I mentioned to the scheduler that I have this itching, which changes everything. She tells me I need a diagnostic mammogram, which requires a doctor's order. They need to spend more time with me and take more pictures. Oh, goodie.

I don't have time for this, was my thought. The holidays were fast approaching and there was simply too much shopping in my future, among other things. All this fuss over nothing, was my view.

Being the good girl that I am, I made the call and obtained the order and the appointment. Knowing this was nothing I scheduled work appointments later that day, as this was merely a formality. And besides the itching was gone.

I love how they tell you to hold your

breath for the mammogram picture.

Just who in the world can breathe

in those things anyway?

If you've never had a mammogram, don't worry—they really aren't that bad. There are too many horror stories floating about and the truth is this exam is a true lifesaver. Yes, the plastic plates that hold and compress your breast are pretty tight. But this only lasts for a few seconds and the peace of mind that you are healthy is well worth the discomfort. Some women take a bit of ibuprofen an hour before their test.

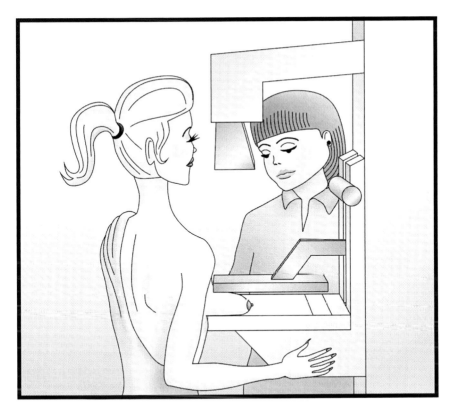

This is what a mammography machine looks like.

When they asked me back to take some more pictures it did not alarm me. I was a very busty Betty and this had happened more often than not. It never occurred to me they had seen something.

Then the mood changed and everyone seemed a lot more serious. Maybe all this extra work has put them behind schedule, I thought to myself. The tech started some small talk, asking me about my home and such things. She seemed nervous. This was interesting to me, as I was sure she'd seen loads of women who didn't pass this test and surely it was routine somewhat by now . . . ? It moved me how despite doing this every day it still affected these professionals. I appreciated their empathy.

She showed me the area in question which looked like lots of tiny polka dots. These polka dots were tiny calcifications which can indicate a change in the breast tissue. When they saw this, they investigated further by taking more pictures. They also compared my current images to my previous mammograms which had been done yearly for ten years at this same breast center. It made things clearer that this is something new.

If you change breast centers, or move to a new city, bring your films.

A historical perspective is very helpful to doctors.

These additional pictures showed a very small area of concern which was my tumor. The radiologist was kind and told me she wanted to do the biopsy right then. I didn't live nearby, so this would spare me a return trip.

When your gut tells you something is up, it usually is.

These ladies weren't fooling me for a minute.

So up on the biopsy table I went. It's a funny, not especially soft, contraption. You lay face down, letting your affected breast hang down through a charming little hole. Oh dear, this is very odd—like a massage table, but really very much not.

The table elevates, not unlike your stylist's chair, and the doctor works from below. They put numbing medicine in the breast first, and then they use a probe to take some tissue.

Tissue? I could use some, thank you! Tears are coming!

Am I dreaming this? This is too bizarre to believe.

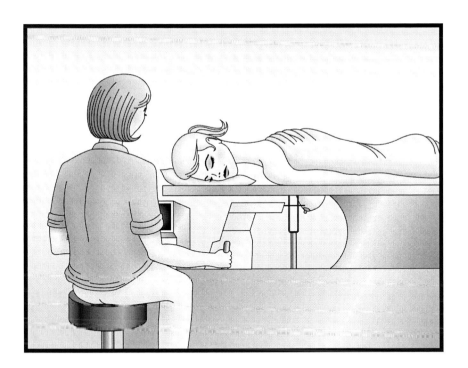

This is what it looks like.

Soon it is all over and you are sitting in a chair recovering while the technician prepares the slides. What my doctor and the nurses did not realize is I know how to read these things, having spent so many years working in radiology as a nurse. The X-Ray image of the tissue sample was on a screen near where I was seated. I could see my cancer looking right back at me. What a strange feeling.

The next day was spent trying to keep myself busy as I waited for the biopsy results. It was a very long day. I already knew the answer. Why wait for a lab to tell me what I already knew? So was the first example of the rules:

Doctors make final decisions based on the lab results.

The final pathology is king.

So the call came. The breast radiologist, though not the same one that did the biopsy, was patient and kind. She gently informed me they had found cancer. Yes, I knew that. Thanks, but no thanks. Crap.

So after I could catch my breath I asked her what the next steps were. She mentioned a breast MRI and then seeing a surgeon. What? I only have this small tumor! Why such a fuss?

That's the funny thing about cancer.

Even the small ones can cause trouble.

I explained to her, in my most convincing demeanor, that all this wasn't neces-sary, and though I appreciated her concern, again, thanks but no thanks. I had made it to forty-seven without having anything major happen concerning my health, and surgery was simply out of the question.

God love her, she stayed with me, and persisted. She didn't give me an out, which for a slippery cat like me was probably the best approach. She explained the two options of lumpectomy and mastectomy. She added that lumpectomy would also require radiation, which is something I wasn't up for, though I knew it is a popular option. I was concerned about what that could do to my body long term.

I was appalled at having only two options. Just how can a girl be forced to choose from so little? This is the new millennium for heaven's sake. How can this be? I think I even asked her, "If this is truly the case, then where is all that research money going?" I found out and benefited from the answer to that question later. There have been wonderful advances in treatments— Sentinel Node Biopsy—sur-vival rates, and overall quality of life for breast cancer patients. More on this in chapter 2. I am not sure I was very polite to this poor doctor.

Doctors who deal with cancer must be

heaven's angels on earth.

All I know is they have a great capacity to understand.

Tumor tissue is graded to assess the pace of its growth. The scale they used for mine was from 1 to 3 This is one of those times where you want to score as low as possible. I was a 2, moderate rate of growth.

The cancer is also given a stage once all the data is in, after all the tests. They typically use a 0 to 4 scale and, again, the lower the number the better. The stage depends on tumor size, whether it has spread, etc. A good source of information is the National Cancer Institute website:

www.cancer.gov/cancertopics/factsheet/Detection/staging.

The tumor tissue is tested for three important elements. These are estrogen, progesterone, and a protein called Her2. They are testing for whether the cancer is receptive to these hormones, which naturally occur in the body. Receptive tumors use these hormones for fuel.

You see, if they are receptive, they can give you medicine that helps to block the food source to further cancer cells in your body. This starves them in a sense. You will hear terminology such as "estrogen/progesterone receptor positive/negative." This is often abbreviated as ER/PR +/-.

Mine was negative/negative. They called it "double negative." They didn't have enough of a sample for the protein test.

All the more reason to take away all the breast tissue, I thought. At least that made sense to me. I wasn't eligible for the medication to help prevent this from coming back. Again, I was only forty-seven years old. And fifty is the new thirty after all.

The Bucket Bed

and Other Fine Pieces of Technology

A few days later it was Halloween, time for my scary breast MRI. I don't especially like cramped spaces, and though I am not technically claustrophobic I wouldn't fight a crowd of women to get the best deals at a good sample sale. Some things are just not worth the trouble.

Let them know if you are claustrophobic

and bring a driver.

They will likely put happy juice in your IV.

They will start an IV and give you contrast dye, which helps to highlight the problem area. They remove the IV as soon as the test is complete.

You ride on this table that goes into this enormous magnet. You cannot wear any metal—no jewelry, nothing. Any metal will be pulled into the magnet or heat up if it is in your body. Tooth fillings are okay.

Tell them if you have any implanted devices of any kind.

This includes that cute little belly button piercing nobody knows about.

Wear pants without metal (no zipper). I found some lovely black designer yoga pants at a ridiculous discount and they went with me everywhere. If you wear these you can keep your bottoms and at least some of your modesty intact.

This may seem like a stretch to say

this is a fashion opportunity.

Even if clothes don't make the patient,

it made things easier for me.

Yoga pants are a must.

This is me having my breast MRI, wearing my yoga pants:

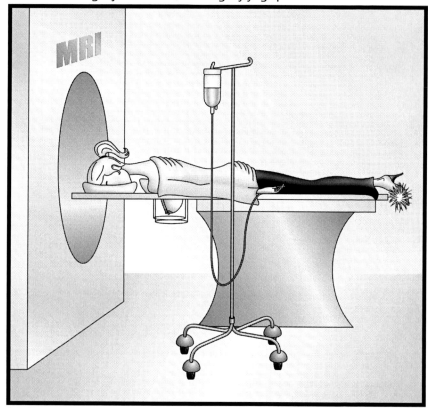

2.1: Breast MRI

The inventor of this must be either the same person who did the biopsy table or at the very least they must have been in the same fraternity. Yes, once again you lay face down, arms at your sides(who sleeps like that?); this time both of your "girls" get to hang in openings in the table.

This must be why they call it the "Bucket Bed."

Your breasts hang in these plastic buckets.

While I appreciate the space program for coming up with this means of taking wonderful pictures, I find it ironic that it originated in a weightless world when gravity seems to be the very key to the body's position. I don't know, but honestly, gravity hasn't been my friend for a while now.

Anyway, the machine is very loud and the sound, though I expected it, startled me every time. There is no pain as it is just pictures, but the table itself isn't all that comfortable. As many places on my body that have extra padding, my sternum is not one of them. Lying there for forty-five minutes made me a bit stiff also, which made the young tech's request afterward for me to "just jump right up" not all that amusing.

Maybe she thought I looked young and fit?

These ladies are just trying to be cheerful.

The next brush with big technology was the PET scanner. It is a scan that uses sugar (now that is certainly something my body is familiar with) to detect cancer cells; a CT machine takes the photos.

They limit your diet a few days prior to the scan and they inject this sugary substance into your IV. I could taste it, which was weird but common they said.

You then are told to relax in this dark room for an hour while this substance spreads throughout your body. I was nervous, but luckily I kept a favorite song in my mind, and the image of my dear college friend singing it. This helped me make it through the hour-long wait. Bring your iPod.

Music is the peacemaker of the soul.

Enjoy as much of it as you can.

The rest of the scan was uneventful. Finally, I was able to lie on my back. Twenty minutes later it was done. They did position my arms over my head for this test. A diagram of this machine is shown on the following page.

If you need a PET scan, do it before your mastectomy.

It will be quite a challenge to raise your arms for a while.

Just before surgery, whether you decide on a lumpectomy or mastectomy, they will want to do what is called the "Sentinel Node injection procedure." This is where they use a substance that shows them the first lymph node the breast drains into, so they can remove just that node and test it to see if the cancer has spread. If negative, they don't have to remove many, if any, additional nodes.

The important point about nodes is a condition called "lymphedema" (pronounced LIMF-eh-DEE-ma). This is when your arm can't empty itself of fluid because it no longer functions properly. It can cause subtle swelling or it can be really serious—and it can be worse than any puffiness you have ever had, believe me.

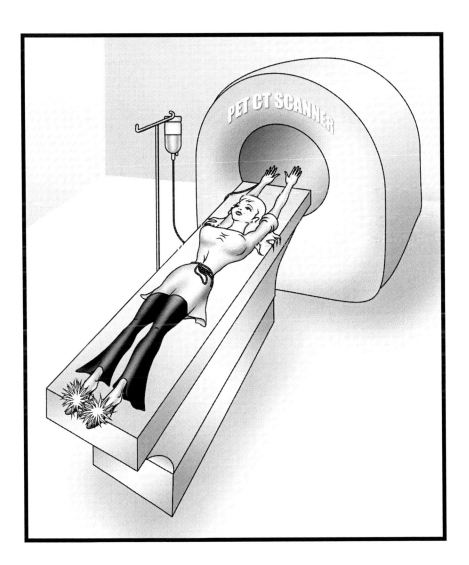

Make sure they measure your arm in several places before surgery.

This will help in detecting swelling moving forward.

Contact a good physical rehab center if

your doctor doesn't offer this.

The doctor will numb your nipple's areola first with a local anesthetic, and then inject a substance that travels through your breast's lymph system. This was very scary for me. It didn't hurt that much. It was more the idea of it, I think.

You need to be a brave lady here

because it is worth the trouble.

This can make a big difference

in your long-term recovery.

Again I remembered my music, only in a very different way. My heart was racing and so was the melody.

Did you know that even hymns, when sung at a very rapid pace,

can sound like rap music?

I don't like rap music.

Then they do a scan and mark the skin above the breast with a felt-tipped pen. This helps the surgeon find the lymph node plus it has a little bit of radioactive stuff in it that lights up their Geiger counter to ensure it is the right one.

This is a huge advance in breast cancer treatment.

This is where a portion of all that money from the pink ribbons went.

All the rest of this, of course, happens when you are fast asleep. And that is just one of life's little blessings. Some parties are just better skipped.

These are the tests I experienced. There are more available and please ask questions so you are as prepared as you can be. Ask for diagrams or a simple drawing of what to expect.

Medical people forget you are so much in the dark.

They are always willing to explain things.

Fight or Flight

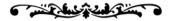

The 603 to Cayman

This was the most surprising thing for me. The mind games my psyche chose to employ were simply amazing. I think my mind was protecting me from taking all of this in at once. It's just too big.

Accepting a cancer diagnosis is like eating a very large apple.

Best to do it in small bites.

"Fight or flight" is medical terminology for the body's response to stress. The body either prepares to combat the enemy or to get the heck out of there as soon as possible. Either way the adrenaline is flowing at a high rate.

My mind gave me this great idea to flee, all right—to a tropical beach where nobody knows me or could find me. It told me if I wasn't me, then I don't have cancer. And if I can't be located, then I don't have to have any treatment. My own witness protection program.

Crazy, huh? Well that's not all. When I looked at the paperwork with my label on it my mind refused to accept that it was for me. I remember sitting in the surgeon's exam room and thinking to myself, Gee, that girl has my same name. Someone needs to get in touch with her right away. She's in trouble.

And, even further detached, I made a mental note of the font the hospital used for these labels, which I rather liked. Again, it was as if I was merely a spectator in this string of events. This happens to other people I have known, not to me. There's never been any cancer in my immediate family. This can't be right . . . can it?

I tried to convince my breast surgeon there was some mistake.

She wasn't taking the bait. Smart lady.

I did end up having genetic testing for the breast cancer gene and the results came back negative. So many people think this is mainly a familial disease, but that is just not true.

The vast majority of breast cancer is not genetic.

Nobody is immune and everyone needs regular mammograms.

The point here is to have regular screenings and to pay attention to your body. Do your monthly breast self-examination. Don't take chances and don't allow your loved ones to either. This is a lifesaving decision; although, like me, this will never happen to you or your dear ones. That is what we tell ourselves anyway.

Men can also get breast cancer, so be sure to have any lump on the males in your life checked out by a doctor.

Early detection is the key.

It saved my life.

These Doctor People:

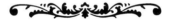

Your Makeover Team

I have never been a gambler, but in this experience I really did feel like I'd won the lottery. At least when it came to my team of doctors that came together to complete this incredible makeover.

As I came to accept this fate, and especially because I was steadfast on my decision for this course of treatment, finding the right doctors became my first priority.

Talk about a *shopping expedition!*

Be choosy. These people need to feel right.

My breast surgeon, Dr. S., was a self-assured lady who showed me I could accomplish what I set out to do, which was to take a bad situation and make the most of it. I am a champion at second-guessing myself, and an all-star worry wart. Doing a double mastectomy was the only logical choice for me. And she respected that.

What happened in that exam room was nothing short of magic. I came in a terrified child and through her kind words and reassuring, confident manner, I emerged an empowered woman. I knew what I wanted and had the right person to do the job. I was going to be free of this cancer and lovely to boot.

Dr. S. even tracked me down at quite a late hour on a Friday night, on a holiday weekend no less, to give me my final pathology results. We had all been anxiously awaiting them and she understood and respected that.

My first experience with a plastic surgeon wasn't as wonderful. He was cool and aloof, and it really bothered me how he ran his fingers through his hair all the time. Now I love hair, and his was lovely, but it tends to be kind of dirty, I think, and there is a reason for all those hair nets.

It just wasn't a good fit. He wanted me to wait, as much as a year, to be sure I wasn't going to need chemo or radiation, as this would interfere with his treatment schedule. I couldn't believe what I was hearing. He expected me to be without "the girls" for a year? What?

Your plastic surgeon needs to be wonderful.

You will spend a great deal of time with this person.

So I called the breast center and told them to try again. Meanwhile I started asking around and both a friend and a lab worker at my home clinic told me about this wonderful guy who also plays in a band. I love music more than most. Maybe there is something to this. How could two very different people refer me to the same doctor?

There are no coincidences in life.

Just angels spreading their magic to make things happen.

The clinic called to say they had another surgeon for me to meet and he, oddly enough, sounded very much like the name I was about to request. He was one and the same. I knew this was meant to be. Funny thing is, I ended up mispronouncing his name for months. He never corrected me. He was really considerate on all levels.

Our first meeting was really emotional for me, as he wanted to be certain I was sure about my decision to have all this surgery. It is a year-long process, he explained: Four surgeries in all and a lot of appointments. A true life interruption for a year.

This is not an easy road. There are many steps to take.

For me it was worth every one.

Now, who doesn't love plastic? A good credit card can get a gal through many a difficult spot. A great plastic surgeon can carry you through a dark time when fear tries to cloud the landscape leaving you feeling lost and alone.

The divine Dr. M. did this for me. He understood what I wanted to do and why. He said he'd be there for me and he was. I have never seen such compassion in a doctor. It was truly genuine. Honestly, it blew me away

Take a good look at photos of their patients before and after.

A picture really is worth a thousand words.

Later I attended a focus group of breast cancer patients. This was my first exposure to a group of survivors. Most were one to two years out or more. I was four months. They were still reeling from the struggles they experienced. I felt really pretty good. Then it occurred to me what the difference was.

None of them had reconstructive surgery.

They were missing the "M Factor."

I took it as my own personal research observation. Women who do not wake up from mastectomy with new "breasts" suffer a lot more than those of us who did. Women who don't have the light of a great plastic surgeon to lead them out of their dark days are at a great disadvantage. At least it seemed that way to me.

The "breasts" I woke up with were temporary and were used to prepare my body for the eventual implants. I called these my spacers/rocks. More details on these in chapter 15.

There are many doctors that will contribute to your care.

Chances are at least one of them will be divine.

My first oncologist visit didn't go well. A friend recommended him and I was happy to meet him. I wasn't happy to sit in a very sad waiting room filled with really sick people. My heart bled for them. Worse yet, this doctor thought it was appropriate to be funny when I was really scared.

Cancer offices can be scary and sad places, especially the first time.

Bring a friend to support and distract you.

When we disagreed on my course of treatment things just went from bad to worse. He was sure I needed chemo because my tumor was double negative. Sorry, not in my plan. Not unless absolutely necessary.

As much as chemotherapy can be very effective, all medications have side effects and I was not excited to experience any of them. I don't even like to take aspirin unless I really need it. A second opinion regarding this type of treatment is advisable. Doctors are accustomed to this and you need the best care. You deserve peace of mind. Don't be concerned about anyone but yourself right now.

My mistake here was not to ask for another oncologist right then and there. I somehow thought he would grow on me as he came so highly recommended. I should have talked to someone else. This would have saved me a lot of emotional pain. I went for a month thinking I had to have chemo, regardless of the fact my tumor was tiny and hadn't spread.

If you doubt your doctor's recommendation, get another.

This is too important to be unsure.

I was referred to another oncologist whom I met after my surgery. His name was PJ and I thought this was the perfect nickname for someone who made me feel as comfy as my pajamas do.

Kind, patient, and incredibly intelligent, he was the perfect match. I am so glad to have made the switch. It is really important to feel confident and well cared for.

If your doctor doesn't feel like a good fit, find another.

There is no shame in this.

Checking your doctor's credentials is a good idea. Ask them how many of these procedures they have done. And if they are board certified. There are ratings on physicians on the web, some are free while others require a small fee. A friend checked this for me. Also, I asked around the breast center and community.

My new oncologist agreed with what the surgeons had predicted and I never had to do chemo. Then the first oncologist revisited my case and agreed with this also.

Another very important element to my care was the insurance company. I had heard and read of the many struggles other women had endured trying to get their procedures approved and funded.

It is bad enough that you are in the fight for your life.

You shouldn't have to battle the insurance company.

I called mine and asked for validation on what was allowed and what was to be paid by them. I also reviewed what I would be expected to pay.

Of particular concern to me was the removal of a healthy breast. My friend had trouble getting her insurance company to approve this. I shared this concern with my breast surgeon, Dr. S., and she assured me this would not be an issue and it wasn't. This is just another reason I felt so wonderfully cared for.

In the U.S. there is a federal law regarding

breast cancer surgery.

If your insurance funds mastectomy,

they must also fund reconstruction.

Visit this site for more information:
www.dol.gov/dol/topic/health-plans/womens.htm

It is very helpful to keep a running list in a notebook of all the various medical bills you will receive. My insurance company sent a monthly statement, which I used to simply check them off one by one as they were paid. Most insurance companies do not provide these.

You can likely view your bills online but there is no organized statement that allows you to keep track yourself. This notebook will save you a lot of confusion and grant you some peace of mind in a most difficult time.

A great inexpensive binder, "Cancer 101," made specifically for cancer patients to help organize everything, can be ordered at www.cancer101.org/planner.

Hospitals have financial counselors that can help you with setting up payment terms if you cannot pay your bills all at once. They may also have resources to refer you to for assistance. Call and ask for the accounting department.

Find Your Amy

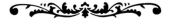

This person is essential to your support system and to organizing all the many pieces of information that make up this process. They attend your doctor visits with you, take notes (when you are so freaked out you can't hear a word that is told to you), and give you invaluable opinions.

I am so lucky to have my wonderful, loving sister Amy who was right there with me during all my many visits to help me digest and decipher all the information. Her support was a rock I could hold on to when the waters got rough. And having that second set of eyes and ears was so helpful.

You really need this person. A friend, neighbor—someone.

Husbands are not always the best choice.

Men can be so uncomfortable with the whole breast subject matter, in a clinical setting anyway. And spouses are pretty scared already.

Amy and I talked for hours about what we heard and understood, and she helped communicate with the rest of the family. She giggled with me when I wanted to and cried with me when I needed that.

We even picked out my new breasts at a Greek restaurant after an appointment, from a lovely statue of Aphrodite. Now that is a shopping experience I never saw coming.

Find Your Betsy

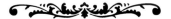

Betsy is a dear friend and coworker with whom I only have the privilege of seeing once a year at our annual meeting. Delightful, pretty as a picture, I always look forward to seeing her. Only last year our conversation was a surprising one.

She had recently been diagnosed with breast cancer and was in the midst of her reconstruction. I was amazed at her attitude, as she was so optimistic. I was spellbound by her story and she was more than happy to explain it all to me. I remember feeling honored that she was so open. I was sure this information would help someone I knew some day.

So when that person turned out to be me, Betsy was one of the first people I called. She instinctively knew why I needed her. This began the guidance I would quickly grow to rely on in the coming days, weeks, months.

Truly, she was indispensable. She was the only person who could tell me exactly what to expect and answer the many questions that raced through my mind. It is so different hearing a fellow patient's point of view.

Ask to talk to someone who's been in your shoes.

They are the only ones that really know.

Reach to Recovery (www.reachtorecovery.org) is a large group of survivors who have agreed to assist newly diagnosed patients with phone support and a listening ear. Some breast centers have their own group they use.

They say it's a club you never asked to join; yet Betsy assured me I would have the opportunity to pay it forward and soon. She was right about that. Helping other women has been some of the most rewarding work of my life.

My friend Deb was an executive at the breast center and she introduced me to the manager. Carol was so patient and kind to me, supportive of my treatment decision, and very respectful. She was also so knowledgeable. I felt lucky to have the chance to meet her.

Surprisingly, this meeting gave me a chance to offer some solutions to things that could make things easier for patients in the breast care program. Carol was always happy to hear my ideas and I hope in some small way these ideas helped other women.

Don't assume your ideas have been thought of.

Sometimes the best ones are the easiest.

A friend who was diagnosed a month before me chose to have a lumpectomy for her treatment, which left her affected breast one full cup size smaller than the other. There are many choices in prosthetic devices and custom bra options, but these can be pretty costly. Her insurance didn't cover this, but many plans do.

I decided to find some of those really heavily padded bras on clearance in her pre-surgery size and removed the padding with a scissors on her unaffected side. The padding filled in her smaller breast and the bra fit normally on the other one. She was now completely symmetrical in her clothing. Rather than a fifty-dollar solution, I found something that worked great for five dollars. What a thrill for both of us.

Cry, Baby:

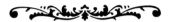

The Pink Raccoon

If fear is the foundation of a cancer diagnosis, then tears are the price of admission.

My sister Julie warned me about the freight train. I believed her, knowing she had experienced it more than once, but didn't expect it to hit with such force. Silly I suppose, as the phrase itself implies just that.

As much of a challenge the physical side of this experience can be, the emotional side is the real test. I remember Dr. M. telling me this. For whatever reason my brain could not rule out the possibility of dying, which in my early stage of the disease was simply not going to happen.

But true to emotions, they are not often logical. A lot of my cancer sisters had the same feeling. Do not pass go, do not collect your two hundred dollars. Take the next flight to the sky.

Facing this ultimate truth is not necessarily a bad thing.

It reminds you of how wonderful your life is.

The important thing is to let it out. Cry as much as you want to, as much as you need to. Go to the mountaintop and let out your best primal scream. Do whatever you need to do to process the feelings of fear.

Bottling the feelings up inside can be

a very, very bad idea.

You could end up hurting someone you love.

My mother suggested I pace myself. She knew the difficulty of illness first hand. She said there would be times when it was difficult to think past the present to the next day. Taking it one day, even one hour at a time is a good way of coping. I found this to be true and quite helpful at a few points in this process.

It's been a year from my diagnosis and I still cry. Just not nearly as often and not in public as I used to. It's more under control now. This will be the same for you, too, in time.

Hang in there, my sister.

This will get better.

I cried so much in the hospital while awaiting my final pathology test (shows the doctors the actual size of the tumor and if it matches what the other tests showed) that the tender skin on my Scandinavian face (under my eyes) was pink and chapped. I tried to think of how to heal it and nothing helped.

I called this the Pink Raccoon.

Turns out that old-fashioned, first-aid cream

healed it overnight.

But not before my dear mother saw me. The sight of it broke her heart. I am so sorry that happened. She's a smart cookie, and regardless of how strong I was in front of her, I know she was scared. And she knew I was.

One thing you can tell your friends and family, as well as your doctors, is that touching a breast cancer patient is okay. No, it's more than okay, it's vital. And a hug can be a hug, not too tight, but a real hug anyway. I was lucky to have lots of these.

These half hugs simply have to go.

I also found that a very useful tool in getting me prepared for the events to come was anger. Yes, I got good and mad. How could this disease just show up unannounced and uninvited? Where were its manners for goodness' sake?

Getting mad helps strengthen you

against your enemy: cancer.

Remember, it's that which you're fighting, not your caregivers.

If you can't get angry, then look at this way. You would do anything to protect your child/niece/pet—you are fighting to protect their mother/aunt/master. What could be more important?

So get tough and fight like mad.

Fight like a girl.

It helps to transform you from a victim into a fighter. And remember . . .

You are stronger than you think you are.

You can do this.

Soul Sisters and Brothers

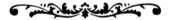

Family is one of life's greatest blessings, and when I was faced with this challenge I was so grateful for the strength and support of mine. They were always there for me—checking in, supporting me. I knew I had my helpers squarely in position for whatever I needed.

Their reaction was of no surprise to me. I have always known a great sense of family and have myself been the supporter when needed. There is not much in this world that matters more than this, at least not to me.

My sister Nancy lives some six hundred miles away and wanted to express her gratitude to Dr. M. for all his wonderful support. This meant so much to her, as she couldn't be with me in person. She sent a lovely card and note that touched him. This was such a nice gesture that we both appreciated.

There are evidently some life events that tend to blur the lines of blood and water. My friends were also wonderful to me. I was rarely without someone to call, if only to pass the time and try to normalize things. They called often to check in on me and to share support and encouragement.

What was important to me regarding my circle of support was to be open and honest with them, and this being the basis of my personality it was no stretch. Everyone is intelligent and wanted to learn as much as I was willing to share.

Something I learned from a cancer sister was to understand the need for my circle to be able to help me.

Be sure to ask for help with things you

won't be able to do for a while.

It helps your dear ones with their coping and healing.

I needed help with drivers to appointments, as they won't let you operate heavy machinery while on painkillers. I needed people to distract me from the consuming subject at hand. A lot of the time, I just needed to talk.

Many friends and family lifted me up in prayer. I was amazed by the sheer volume of support. Six church congregations, at least. The doctors were not acting alone. This was going to turn out really well.

It can be very difficult to see

your dear ones afraid for you.

I spent a lot of my time trying

to convince them I was fine.

The funny thing about this is when you spend so much effort doing so, it just naturally tends to rub off on you. You start to really believe it. When you consider that outcome, positive thinking really does help promote a good chain of events.

A message to family and friends: the patient knows you are scared. The truth is there isn't much she can do about that but to accept it as a sign of love and caring. Staying strong is key, as the patient is in a crisis and should not have to deal with everyone else's issues. Don't make this about yourself. Just listen and support the patient.

My brother Bruce told me he wasn't worried because I told him not to be. I was touched by how well he listened and tried to pretend for my sake.

Scared Hubby

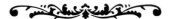

In sickness and in health, to love and to cherish. These vows can't prepare either one of you for a serious illness. Not that anything really can. I have read where cancer can bring couples closer. We were already as one. It just scared us both a great deal.

My dear husband was there for me at every turn. We talked for hours when I couldn't sleep. He held my hand and wiped my tears. Yet there were times he needed to be alone in his garage shop. I didn't always understand why.

Everyone copes with things in a different way.

Some need to be alone.

It is important to remember this

so it isn't misunderstood.

I should have remembered this from living with my dear dad. He tends to work when faced with adversity. I have seen him chop a whole lot of wood over the years.

The hardest part for us was I was pretty sore after the biopsy and subsequent exams. My husband knew this and didn't want to cause me any more discomfort. I needed to be held. The two things were mutually exclusive.

The physical and emotional struggle can often be linked.

Try to find a means of communicating what you need.

The loss of sleep only makes everything worse. My emotions were even more raw.

The change in my body was an adjustment for both of us. My husband was very understanding and respected my need to transform what I thought was a figure flaw while also decreasing the chances of the cancer returning.

It's sad how women are so critical regarding their bodies.

Men have told me there is no such thing as ugly breasts.

I am happy to report we are both quite pleased with my new look. We see this as our silver lining. Getting our groove back in the bedroom took some time but healing, acceptance, and love is a powerful combination.

You may not have a spouse or significant other. I ask you to reach out to a sibling or friend, as this support is vital to your recovery. Sometimes family can retreat as a means of coping, so looking beyond your immediate circle may be necessary.

There are many resources to tap into online; ask about this where you have your mammogram. There are also a lot of chat rooms online that can be supportive. If you aren't comfortable using a computer, ask someone to help you. This is a great idea for children or grandchildren, as they excel at this and would likely feel happy to help you in some way.

Puppy Love

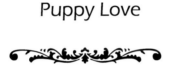

Man's best friend is named Winston Churchill in our home. He is a poodle mix and as smart as they come, maybe smarter. He loves both of us very much, but can appear to favor me at times.

He is ten years old now and not nearly as affectionate as he was as a puppy. Yet, when cancer entered our family he never left my side. He even sat next to me in the powder room. He was and continues to be a great support to me.

This may sound crazy, as this

diagnosis upends your life as it is.

But, I think you really need a loving dog.

I don't mean to say this is a decision to be made lightly, of course. It is a big commitment. I just know how much unconditional love my puppy brought into our family and extended family. I am thinking this could be really powerful medicine. Maybe find a friend with a puppy or visit your local Humane Society for some cuddle time.

My darling niece Kelly's first word was doggie. She has always understood the love of a dog. I gave her a little white poodle stuffed animal as a gift when she was a baby.

Her mommy, my sister Amy, was heading over to the hospital to see me after my mastectomy. Kelly went to her room, grabbed the poodle toy, and gave it to her mommy to give to me so I wouldn't be so scared. She was only three.

Later when I was able to return the toy to Kelly, and thanked her for thoughtfulness, she had some questions for me. She asked:

"Were you sick?" I said yes.

"Why?" I said I didn't know.

"Were you scared?" I said yes.

"Did you cry?" I honestly replied yes.

She then put her little head down and said, "I'm sorry."

We hugged and I assured her I was okay. I will always remember this gesture of selfless compassion from my sweet, tiny little niece.

Beautiful moments come at unexpected times.

Celebrate them for what they are.

Honestly, as many times that my heart ached during this process, this made me feel like mine was suddenly too big to be contained within my body.

Find Your Susan

My dearest friend Susan was in disbelief like me at the news. We share each other's joy and pain so for her this was particularly difficult.

But true to the strength of a fellow glamour girl she quickly sprang into action. First, she went to the local bookstore in search of information. She mailed me four books on breast cancer, three of which I read in the first week.

She knew I needed to understand what was happening to help me cope with the volumes of information, appointments, and emotional upheaval. Your mind doesn't have the ability to absorb it all at once.

Your Susan will know what you need.

Reach out to her.

She listened to me and was always there for me. She made a list of what I should bring to the hospital and sent it along with one of her many letters. She coached me on the importance of writing down my questions so I was organized for my doctor visits. It helps to keep all of your notes in one journal, and be sure to ask the people who join you to the hospital to take notes when you know your own notes will be unclear. Write down the date and name(s) of person(s) you spoke to, along with their phone number(s).

Write a list of questions for the doctors.

You will have several caregivers and this helps organize things.

It was funny for me that I would need such a list, as I am medically educated. But I did, as my emotional state did a number on my ability to get my thoughts across. I found this maddening even though I understood it to be perfectly normal.

Susan lives in Texas so she had to fly to my city to be with me for the surgery. She was glad to come and made it easy for me to accept her help.

I remember seeing her standing at the airport curb. We aren't typically very emotional with each other but when I saw her, I ran to her. We wept in each other's arms. It was so good to see my dear friend.

Cancer changes the way you react to things.

Some are for the better.

So, after a quick stop for a latte, we headed straight to the wig shop. Susan didn't skip a beat when I asked her if this was okay. She knew that I needed her help in choosing something that would help me look my best.

That's when we met Rita. She was so patient and understanding. I tried many styles and eventually chose a darling chin-length bob in the same blonde as my "natural" hair color. It was amazingly authentic-looking for synthetic hair.

So this is how I finally had the chance to look like a doll.

What a strange way that came about!

Honestly, the wig looked better than my real hair. A lot of that was because when stressed or sick my hair lies flat. This was a huge boost for me and it came at just the right time. Surgery was the next day. You see, at this point I was still under the impression I needed chemo, regardless of my early stage of the disease.

Losing my hair was going to be one of the most difficult parts of this journey, at least for a glamour girl like me.

Rita offered to put it on hold until I received my final diagnosis, saying some people end up receiving good news and do not need the wig. I appreciated that comment but at the time didn't think it would end up applying to me.

When it did, I chose to pay it forward—I funded a wig for my good friend who was going through treatment at another facility and had not found anything. I called the wig store to give them my credit card number and then directed my friend to the salon. I asked Rita to stand strong and refuse her money.

That worked out really well. For all the many things my friend has done for me over the years, this was my chance to do something for her. And to surprise her was even better. Her insurance didn't adequately cover wigs, though many do.

She called me quite jubilant at her new hairdo. Tired of the scarves and the unwanted attention, this gave her an ability to be social.

When you are having a bad time of things,

help someone else.

It is a high you will not soon forget.

It still makes me smile.

Susan stayed with me before and after my surgery, along with my sister Amy and my husband. She slept in my room and helped me through that first night. Actually, she didn't really sleep much at all.

She was summoned back to Texas that next day due to a family emergency. I know she feels like she let me down but that is so far from the truth. I felt her with me always and neither time nor distance could ever change that.

Feather Your Nest:

Shopping!

There are some items you will need to make this experience easier. These are easily found at your favorite department or discount store.

A little pampering goes a long way

in the midst of all this.

Treat yourself to some lovely things.

As the mastectomy will limit your arm movement for a time, you are best to look for a few sets of front-buttoned pajamas. Raising your arms to don a pullover of any sort will be a challenge for a while.

I found some great knit pajamas on sale,

which were especially soft.

I also found some silkier options for wearing at home.

Fuzzy socks are great also. This is something your friends or family can provide if they want to help. They are not expensive and are really a sweet gift.

You will also need button- or zip-front tops for doctor visits. These are easy to wear with your yoga pants. Just remember, nothing that goes over the head.

Something I found to be essential is camisoles. You will not be wearing a bra for several months while awaiting your implants. These helped me to feel covered and supported, as well as feminine.

You will need two different types of

camisoles or tank tops:

several inexpensive ones right

away and pretty ones for later.

My thought was to not spend much on the ones that would likely become stained right after the surgery. I tossed these after they were no longer needed. Inexpensive stretchy tank tops work well.

Here is a list of things I put together ahead of time:

- Extra pillows and pillowcases

- Camisoles, plain and fancy

- Button-front pajamas

- Slippers and fuzzy socks

- Zip- or button-front tops for doctor visits

- Magazines and catalogs

- Chic flicks

- Gentle laxative

The pain medications you will take tend to cause some pretty significant constipation. Betsy recommended I take a gentle powdered laxative for three days prior to my surgery and it kept things moving afterward a breeze. You don't need to suffer constipation on top of everything else.

My surgery was just before Thanksgiving so I needed to get my holiday shopping done before then. I was able to wrap the gifts after surgery, but was glad to have them already at home. Thinking ahead to your temporary limited independence can be a big help in preparing for it.

Hospital Days:

It's No Spa

My caregivers at the hospital were really terrific. I was eager to get the surgery done and they were amazed at my determination. The best part about this was my physical body carried this forward and recovered quickly, as my mind was doing a lot of sleeping.

The mind and body are as one.

Do your best to think yourself well.

My pain control really wasn't a struggle, as long as I informed the nurses in time. This is important to remember even after you return home.

Don't be a hero. Stay ahead of the pain.

Ask for something when it is still early.

Another good trick is to remember to breathe deeply. This relaxes your muscles and can really affect your level of pain. Dr. M. suggested a yoga breathing technique and was with me when I first tried it. It worked, and I couldn't believe it.

Take slow, deep breaths through your nose.

Exhale through your mouth. Repeat.

Another very important breathing technique is called the "incentive spirometer." If the nursing staff doesn't give you one, ask for this. You will need to keep your lungs inflated and healthy as you are spending too much time in bed. This helps prevent pneumonia and other problems.

Use your spirometer often, maybe once an hour.

Try to do ten deep breaths.

Drinking a lot of water is also good to flush the anesthetic and other things out of your body. This was no problem for me, as I woke up really thirsty.

Don't try to get up to the bathroom by yourself, as you will be very dizzy, even after the first day or two. Falling is a danger and, remember, you can't use your arms to break the fall. You don't want to untie all that fancy embroidery.

Walking with help is a very good idea.

It helps to get your strength back

and you will feel a lot better.

Your lips will likely be very dry due to the medications. Use a lot of lip balm or ointment often to avoid the hassle of chapped lips.

Your throat might be sore from the breathing tube they use during surgery. Have your family find you some lozenges to cool this.

Don't expect to sleep much the first night. There are machines for your blood pressure, IV pumps, and other things that all make noise. This gets better quickly as you progress toward being able to go home. If you like these, ask if you can bring a white noise machine to soothe your environment.

Treat the nurses well as they genuinely want to help you feel better. I decided to buy some chocolates for them just before my surgery so my husband could give them to the staff without having to go out and buy them. They really appreciated this.

I was lucky to receive three flower bouquets during my stay. I thought about taking them home but decided it was a better idea to share them.

Consider giving your flowers to patients

who don't have any.

The nurses are happy to do this.

The bandage will be around your entire chest and will be taken off in the first day or so. Also, you will have drains to collect excess fluids. I will tell you more about these in chapter 15.

My nipples were removed as part of the reduction approach. Some women can keep them, but that depends on the situation. Your plastic surgeon will let you know your options.

There is no pat formula for how many days you will stay in the hospital. I stayed for three days. This brings me to another one of the rules:

Everyone heals at a different pace.

You may hear this a lot from your caregivers.

Here is a list of what you may want to take to the hospital:

- List of phone numbers to call

- Throat lozenges

- Your favorite lotion

- Button-front pajamas and slippers

- Headband or hair clips

- Tinted lip balm

- White noise machine

- Three boxes of candy for the nurses

- Pillow to leave in the car

You may experience bloating after surgery. My robe, which was perfect before surgery, barely fit afterward. In reaction to the operation, my body retained fluid.

The best way to rid yourself of this is to drink lots of water and walk with assistance. Excess fluid will be flushed out of your body by your kidneys and you will be back to your normal proportions very soon. Mine only took a few days to resolve.

Walking, in general, is a great way to stay strong before surgery, though I didn't do this. I wish I had, as the combination of anxiety, stress, and inactivity made me gain twenty pounds during this year-long process. Many of my cancer sisters experienced the same thing.

Taking it off is never easy and it seems the body reacts differently to diet and exercise after experiencing this. You may have to try something new to get back to your former self, or to get to the new fabulous you.

There are many professionals that can help with this—doctors, nutritionists, and physical therapists, to name a few. And always remember to ask your new network of cancer sisters for ideas.

Pillow Talk

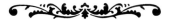

Aside from the love of family and friends, and a few choice medications, I have to say pillows were and continue to be a great source of comfort to me. These are not just the ordinary, flat pillows, mind you, but the fluffy luxurious kind.

I bought three pillows to convert the sofa into a lovely bed, and noticed the nurses used these to help prop up my arms in the hospital, which was really helpful. For the first few months following my surgery, I slept in a reclining position and the flexibility and support of the pillows was essential. My couch was the best option for the first few nights.

Pamper yourself, as these are not expensive.

Remember the soft pillowcases, too.

You will also need a pillow to use in the car for the trip home and other excursions. This should be a firmer pillow; something like an accent pillow for a chair. The firmness holds you snugly under the shoulder strap of the seatbelt.

I bought a fun leopard-print pillow.

I didn't see why it couldn't have a bit of style.

Dangle Earrings and Rocks

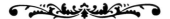

I am really more of a post-style earring girl. These are a very necessary part of the healing process. They are not pretty, nor are they comfortable. And they require care.

This is what they look like, though you will only see part of them.

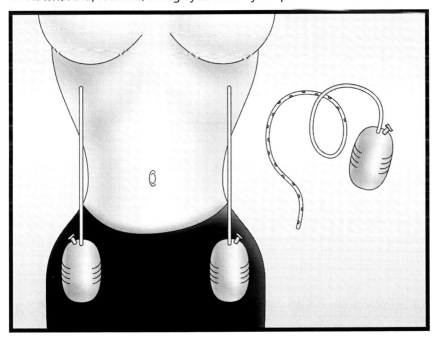

15.1: JP Drains

These are used to drain away the excess fluid in your chest so the tissues can heal. Without them, you may encounter unsightly pockets of stuff in your body that require draining anyway. You will likely not heal properly without them.

These must be emptied a few times a day, or when full. They are nothing but a bulb syringe on a tube that has holes in it. The nurses will teach you and your loved one how to do this. You need to measure it and write it down for the doctor.

The drainage is red, but only because it contains a bit of blood. Remember this is a temporary but necessary thing.

Dr. M. didn't let me shower while I had these in me. There is a risk of infection and nobody wants to face that. My husband gave me sponge baths at the sink, which was really rather nice. I had these in me for one week.

The feeling of a hot washcloth on my back was heaven.

No spa treatment had ever been better.

It is important to support these drains with your hands or with safety pins connected to those cheap camisoles I suggested you buy. If they are inexpensive you won't mind a few pin holes in them. Again, I tossed mine after I was done with this portion of the program.

A diamond is a girl's best friend, some call them "rocks." These are what I like to think of as "diamonds in the rough." Dr. M. calls them rocks with good reason. These are what I called my spacers.

Truthfully, the medical community refers to them as "tissue expanders." They are saline-filled, temporary implants that have a metal "port" in them where the doctor or his nurse can add more saline to grow them over time. They help prepare your body for the implants.

These were put in under my chest (pectoral) muscles while I was in surgery for the mastectomies. The great thing is I woke up with breasts. Small, yes, but breasts all the same. I never had to face the mirror without them. Seeing them without nipples was strange. The suture lines were what I expected but still it was a bit difficult to look at in the beginning.

Dressing was not a challenge, as I still looked feminine. Of course, wearing any kind of a bra was out of the question so soon after the operation. And these "breasts"were self-supporting.

Dr. M. calls them "rocks" because they are so firm.

They aren't especially comfortable.

The procedure to increase their size is done with office visits. "Fills" they are called. Mine weren't too bad. My skin was especially sensitive later on and that was a bit difficult. And the chest muscle aches quite a bit while it is being stretched. I usually had trouble sleeping for a day or two afterward.

The metal ports in these are usually not enough to trip the metal detector at airports, though they might. Your plastic surgeon will give you an identification card that you can show the screening staff if you end up setting the alarm off. This happened to me only once, and not at an airport, but it was really pretty easy to overcome.

My level of skin sensation was highly unusual according to Dr. M. In fact, I never really lost much feeling in my chest at all. They tell me most women experience numbness across their chests, underarms, and back, and regular sensation may or may not come back.

Dr. M. said I am one in a thousand.

I prefer one in a million, but that's just math.

I did and still do have some numbness under my arms. That is a strange feeling, as if you were holding your arms out away from your body. I felt a bit like a little penguin. But I guess penguins are pretty cute. It is getting better all the time, just like the doctor said it would.

When you feel like your new spacers/rocks are the right size for your body, then you can cease the expanding. The greatest thing about this is being able to literally try on your new breasts before buying them. What other surgery lets you do that?

Two of my cancer sisters decided to go larger. They were a B cup and are now a full D. This is common, especially among younger patients, I was told. Everyone must decide this for themselves. I went smaller to a full C, or almost a D. I guess we put the "D" in Diva?

Dog Tired

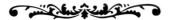

Fatigue is something that comes early in the process and just does not seem to know when to leave. First it is the insomnia that comes from the fear and anxiety of the diagnosis. Later it is from the discomfort of the surgery and the medications that can make you feel strange.

I used over-the-counter medication for sleep, though I was offered more. I didn't see the need to further complicate things dealing with prescription refills when I was doing okay on what I had. Be sure and discuss your ability to sleep or not with your doctor.

Fortunately this is also a temporary condition. I remember the night I was finally able to sleep without help. What a great feeling. It is all part of emerging from this ordeal. It was very liberating.

Ask for help if you can't sleep. This is important.

You need your strength.

Lifting restrictions are standard after surgery, and for a gal on the go like me, this was particularly difficult. The inability to fully use my arms was frustrating yet I truly understood the reasoning behind the order. I wanted my body to heal correctly so I was an angel and followed the directive completely. Not that it was easy.

Someone had warned Dr. M. that I was a go-getter.

Honestly I felt like a dog on a chain.

I found if you ask for help, and prepare your environment prior to surgery, this can be a tolerable situation. I had my husband help with groceries and lifting things around the house. Before my surgery I moved the items I typically use at home down from the cupboards to the counter. I knew that for a time it would be a challenge to reach them.

I also found that using my feet to open heavy drawers and my legs to help me sit up from the sofa was pretty easy.

Necessity truly is the mother of invention.

You will figure out what works for you.

Most women have some sort of physical therapy to help restore the mobility of their arms after surgery. I didn't have to do this. My arm/shoulder movement came back quickly with just routine use.

It is important to exercise your arms on a regular basis, as I can tell even one year later my shoulders would prefer to stiffen up a bit. Some women engage in swimming while others do rowing. Exercise helps to prevent lymphedema also, which is that awful swelling.

Your mind may be a little fuzzy for quite some time after the mastectomy surgery. It was difficult for me to concentrate beyond a few minutes. This steadily improved with time, just a few weeks really, and I was myself again.

The Scrapbook that Wasn't

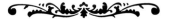

In preparation for my unexpected time off, I put together many things to occupy my time. One of these projects was a small scrapbook I thought might be nice to save the lovely well wishes I was receiving from family and friends. A card is still such a wonderful gesture, maybe even more in this electronic age.

What surprised me was my little scrapbook was nowhere near big enough to hold all the many cards and notes I received. I found a pretty box and kept all of this in there instead. It is something I will always cherish.

If you know someone who needs a lift, send a card.

You never know how much this might help them.

I kept myself busy by keeping up with the many thank-you notes I needed to send for the lovely flowers and gifts sent to me. People were concerned that I should rest and not worry about such things. Honestly, it was good to have this to focus on.

My recovery period began just after Thanksgiving. The presents needed to be wrapped, which was pretty easy for me after a week or two. I also used the time to write out the many Christmas cards we send to friends and family, and to compose a revealing yet hopeful holiday letter.

You can complain that you have so many cards to send.

Or you can be grateful your existence casts such a large net.

Round 2:

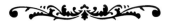

Better than New!

About six months after the first surgery I was ready for the second. I decided to have the silicone implants, as they are much softer than the saline ones and many doctors assured me they were safe. I also read this on the internet. Some doctors may tell you to stay off the internet.

Some of what is on the web is helpful.

Best to ignore the scary stuff and ask your doctor.

To say I was excited for that day is really an understatement. The spacers were pretty uncomfortable by now and I wanted to move on to the next phase of my recovery.

This was a much easier surgery. I was able to go home.

This time without the dangle earrings!

I was pretty swollen for the first week or so, and wondered just how big these things really were. In no time they settled in to the correct shape and size, though my chest was really firm for a while. My muscles were in a bit of a spasm from the surgery. This resolved itself spontaneously.

My implants are very soft and lovely.

They also look very real.

For me this was a new beginning. A chance to have youthful, and more realistic-sized breasts that suited my frame. I can wear so many fashions that were never an option in the past. And the brassiere is now optional.

I don't mean to imply that the loss of a woman's breasts is a trivial thing. I know many cancer sisters grieve this in a significant way. I think I did for a time but came to the conclusion that they were diseased and I really didn't want them any longer. Especially when I saw the reconstructed photographs from Dr. M. For me, beauty and peace of mind were pretty easy to accept. Everyone has to make their own choice.

My recovery was a shortened version of the first time. I used a lot less pain medication and needed less time off work. I was not allowed to lift anything again, not even a little bit. This was more restrictive than the first time. I am sure, again, it was to protect all that elaborate embroidery.

The suture lines you will have depend on the procedure chosen by you and your doctor. I can tell you they do an impressive job at leaving the minimum amount of scarring that will be visible to others. These lines fade with time. It may take a few years until they almost disappear. Of course, this depends on how your body heals.

Here are two examples of suture lines:

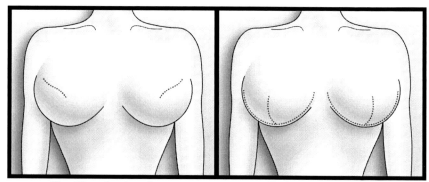

Traditional suture lines.   Reduction approach

My doctor had me wear an underwire bra around the clock twenty-four seven for three weeks (except, of course, in the shower) to help shape my new breasts. He recommended some inexpensive underwire ones, which were fine. Honestly, they gave me support that was comforting during that time. It was odd to sleep with my bra on, but again, this is temporary.

Finishing Touches

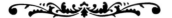

Is it cold in here or is it just me? Headlights, high beams, turkey timers, we've all heard the references. The fact is nipples were an important part of my recovery and my ability to feel whole again.

Once again, I turned to a statue of Aphrodite as a reference. I kept a photo of her in my handbag to show Dr. M. and I experimented in the powder room with those tiny square bandages for placement.

He asked me to wear the bandages the day of surgery (which was about two months after round two) so he would better understand where I wanted these to be placed. I had already planned to do this but it was great to be on the same page as my doctor.

It is important to get your nipples even.

They are always erect.

You see, these don't function like real nipples, even though they are live and have a blood supply. I wanted mine to be small and subtle. Something that on a hot summer day wasn't too obvious under a cute little white top. Remember, wearing a bra is now optional.

My husband pointed out the power these little things can wield. He said he doesn't understand why women are so embarrassed by them.

So stand tall and be proud.

You've earned the right.

Of course, most brassieres have the ability to hide these and that is what I wear on a daily basis. Funny even though the whole bra thing is optional, I still feel more comfortable wearing one. I just don't need the massive support structure of my old ones. I wear comfortable, and very pretty, ones now.

A friend gave me a gift certificate to a

high-end brassiere shop.

A lovely bra is one of the fun things to

add to your new wardrobe.

My surgery for the nipples was an outpatient affair. It wasn't too bad, except for my high level of sensation. The numbing medicine stung.

There are creams on the market

that are used to numb the skin.

These don't work for everybody,

but ask about it if you have sensation.

The suture lines will likely vary by surgeon, but I was surprised at what I found when I was allowed to remove the bandages three days later.

It was more than I expected to see, and that was hard for me. I was feeling a bit like a Halloween pumpkin. Enough carving already. But the suture lines heal and shrink quite a bit. Plus my areola tattoos cover these for the most part.

19.1: Nipple and Sutures

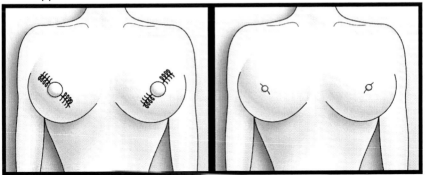

Right after the procedure: After several weeks:

Some women choose to not have the tattoos. Betsy suggested experimenting with semi-permanent lipstick for color and the results were amazingly realistic. I chose a medium bronze color. Send a message to NipColor@gmail.com for more exciting tips on alternatives to tattooing for areola color.

Do not panic. The nipples will be huge for a while.

They need the blood supply to heal. They shrink dramatically.

About 8 weeks after the nipple surgery it was time for the areola tattoos. Finding the right color was important to me. Again, thinking forward to that hot summer day and my cute little white top, I wanted these to also be subtle.

My doctor used a color chart not unlike the hairdresser. I chose almost the lightest color and didn't think to compare it to my skin first. It turned out to be too light. I was nervous about more numbing medicine and wasn't thinking clearly. I can't believe a glamour gal like me missed this.

Be sure to do a color match with the sample to your skin.

Also, remember these tend to fade a bit.

Also, they can be done again if too light.

This was done in the surgeon's office. This time I used the cream and didn't really feel the numbing medicine much at all. The tattoo procedure was easy really. This is good news for me, as I will need to do it over.

I brought a friend along just in case I didn't do well, but we ended up having a lovely lunch and some delightful shopping afterward. She said the transformation from before to after the tattoos was magical. She could not believe how realistic my new breasts were.

19.2 Before and After Tattoo

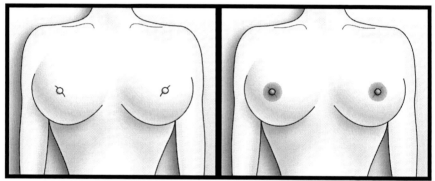

Nipples before tattoo: After tattoo:

Implant revisions are not unusual in the business of breast reconstruction. Even as every procedure is tailored to the specific patient, every human body is unique and heals differently. Medicine truly is as much an art as it is a science in this sense.

Many of my cancer sisters have needed an additional procedure or two in order to achieve the optimal result. I had my right implant replaced to even out my breasts. And my sisters and I can say we are so glad we did. We look fabulous.

I am not suggesting the end result is perfection, as that is not realistic. Yet I am saying the ability to achieve a lovely female form is possible.

Pink is the New Black:

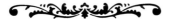

Getting Back to Your Life

When you live and breathe this diagnosis and treatment for a full calendar year it can be difficult to move on. I have read an essential part of healing is to find your way back to your life. Not that this is easy.

This is my one-year cancerversary.

What a difference a year makes.

There are enough pink ribbons to circle the globe, and though well intended, the many references to this became a bit overwhelming. It was as if this was attempting to define me. I didn't want to wear this on my sleeve for the rest of my life. I was going to be healthy again.

That is not to say I fully resisted being a new member of this sorority. I found that helping other newly diagnosed women navigate this maze of a process very rewarding.

Be the pink ribbon lady if it suits you.

Finding how to pay it forward is very fulfilling.

Many women with implants after mastectomy are very open and proud of their "girls." For a lady like me, who is modest to say the least, this was a real stretch. I had flashbacks to the high school locker room where all I wanted to do was hide.

But duty called and I was more than happy to show my new breasts to another sister in peril. I set aside my issues for the greater good. Seeing is believing; and being able to touch (and, yes, massage a bit) the implants on a survivor was key to their understanding of how implants could look and feel. The women were hesitant to ask for this so I volunteered. I knew it was important and would give them optimism.

Not that this was something I was used to.

I haven't had this much action since college.

Of course, every woman needs to be true to themselves in this regard. I chose to help individuals when called upon. To be able to reach out to someone in their darkest days and make a difference is really an amazing feeling. To be able to change someone's tears to laughter and determination is really pure magic to me.

Some friends of mine did the sixty-mile walk. They walked for me and for all the many other people affected by breast cancer. I wasn't up to walking; perhaps I will some day. A friend lit a candle of hope in my honor. I was there in spirit. It was touching how they mentioned me in their efforts.

Let people lift you up as a symbol of hope.

For all women, their daughters, granddaughters,

and all the many people who love them.

I know this is but the beginning of living with cancer, though I don't think of it this way. I am living past cancer. It is a chapter of my life, though quite a challenge, that has given me opportunities to help others while enriching my own. I am not glad it happened but feel making the most of it helps me cope with the reality of it all. It helps me make some sense out of it.

There will be more surgeries as time marches on, as the implants do not last forever. I intend to take each new chapter for what it is, and to embrace the chance to participate in the marvels of modern medicine. I likely will be one of a few women at the senior citizens bingo table with perky breasts. I am perfectly okay with this fact.

Cancer has altered the way I look at things in my life. My priorities have changed. Few things are a tragedy. Many things are more splendid than ever. And I am determined to keep it this way.

Now that I am on the other side of this mountain, I am more alive than ever. It truly is an amazing feeling.

I pray you will find your hope and your strength.

And when you do . . . pass it on.

Helpful Websites

National Cancer Institute

www.cancer.gov

This site offers explanations using simple language with options to email or print fact sheets (in .pdf format) on many subjects pertaining to cancer.

American Cancer Society

www.cancer.org

A great resource for information on all types of cancer.

Susan G. Komen

www.komen.org

To get involved in finding a cure.

Dr. Susan Love

www.armyofwomen.org

For clinical studies.

Cancer planner binder

www.cancer101.org/planner

Reach to Recovery

www.reachtorecovery.org

For survivor support.

Support and stories of hope

www.pinktogether.com

Breast Cancer Organization

www.breastcancer.org

Website for easy-to-understand explanations on all things related to the disease.

To check your doctor's credentials

www.healthgrades.com

American Medical Association

http://webapps.ama-assn.org/doctorfinder

Reports on doctors' records and credentials.

U.S. Dept of Labor

http://www.dol.gov/dol/topic/health-plans/womens.htm

Law regarding reconstruction and insurance.

Glossary of Terms

A fairly simple and straight-forward glossary of breast cancer terms can be found at:

http://www.health-news-aninformation.com/4civista/libv/w19.shtml

For the more scientifically minded, see this technically savvy site:

http://www.cancerlynx.com/breastspore.html

These two sites should cover just about everything on this subject. Of course, being a self-proclaimed "Google Queen," my favorite means of finding information is by conducting searches on the internet, and this almost always works for me.